WELLNESS WEIGH™

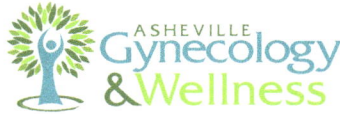

ASHEVILLE
Gynecology
&Wellness

By Dr. Vicky Scott

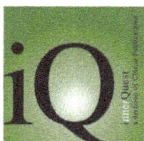

innerQuestBooks.com
ChironPublicatons.com

innerQuest is a book imprint of Chiron Publications
Interior and cover design by Lisa Alford
Printed primarily in the United States of America.

ISBN 978-1-63051-499-0 Paperback
Library of Congress Cataloging-in-Publication Data

Names: Scott, Vicky (Vicky Marie), 1957- author.
Title: Wellness weigh : Asheville gynecology & wellness / by Dr. Vicky Scott.
Description: Ashville, N.C. : Chiron Publications, 2018. | Includes
   bibliographical references and index.
Identifiers: LCCN 2018000492 | ISBN 9781630514990 (pbk. : alk. paper)
Subjects: LCSH: Nutrition. | Health. | Exercise. | Mind and body.
Classification: LCC RA784 .S3916 2018 | DDC 613.2--dc23
LC record available at https://lccn.loc.gov/2018000492

Cover photo by Freepik.

"Let food be thy medicine and medicine be thy food."

~Hippocrates

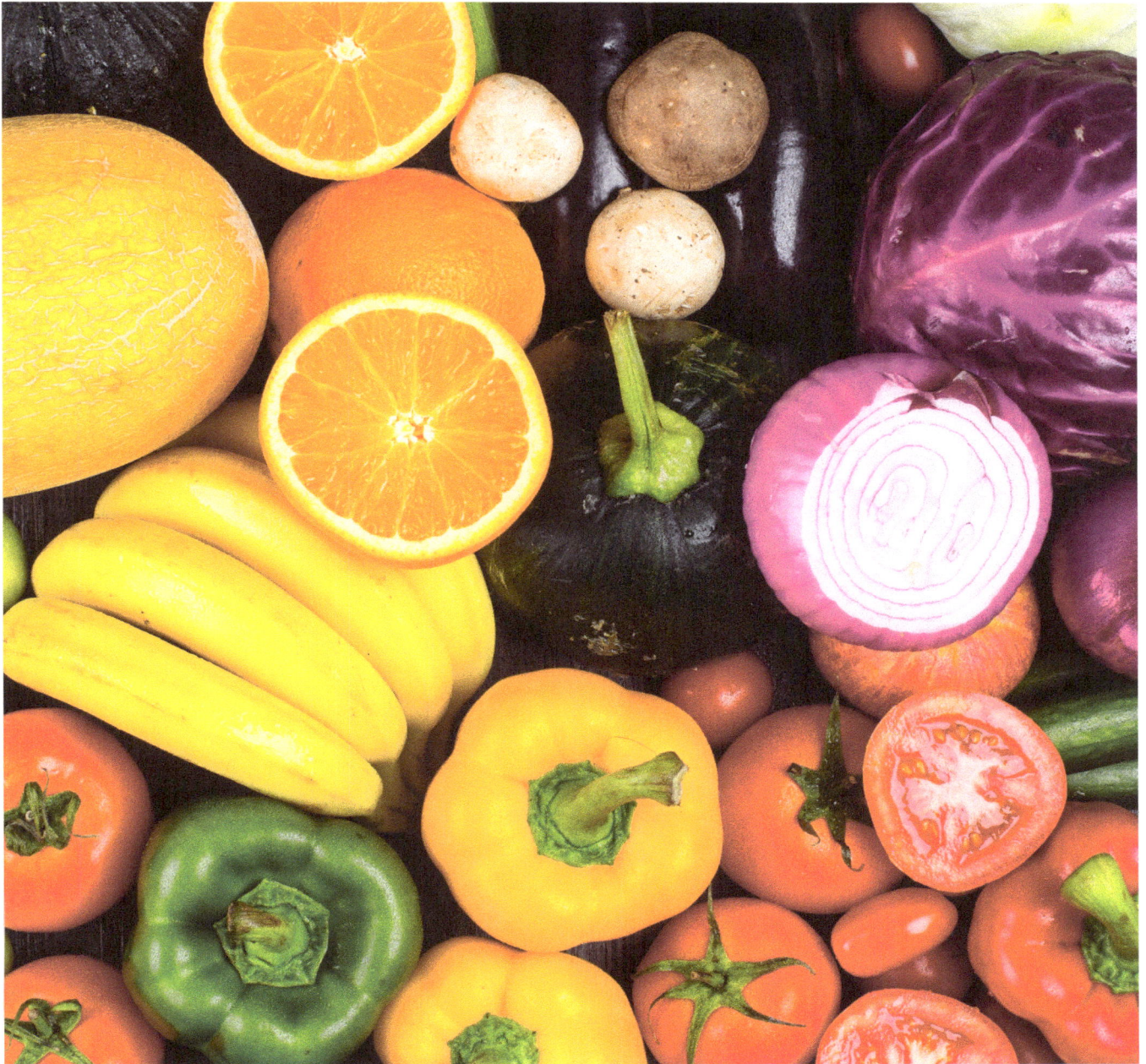

WELCOME

Welcome to your 12-week Wellness Weigh™ program. Our desire is to help you create an attainable goal and to help guide you on a path of self-discovery and empowerment.

Whole Food Plant Based (WFPB) eating provides your body with the nutrients it needs and supports you in making changes that will improve your health. The mind-body-spirit approach encourages you to experience the transition that will occur during your 12-week program on a different level—we hope it will broaden your understanding of what food and wellness means to you.

This booklet is intended to be used as a journal, a log, a guide, or simply an historical record of your journey.

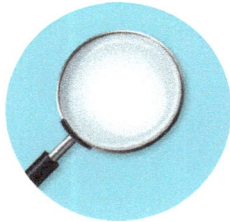

You are encouraged to write reflections on a weekly basis— this will help you embrace focus points presented each week. There is space provided for you to journal.

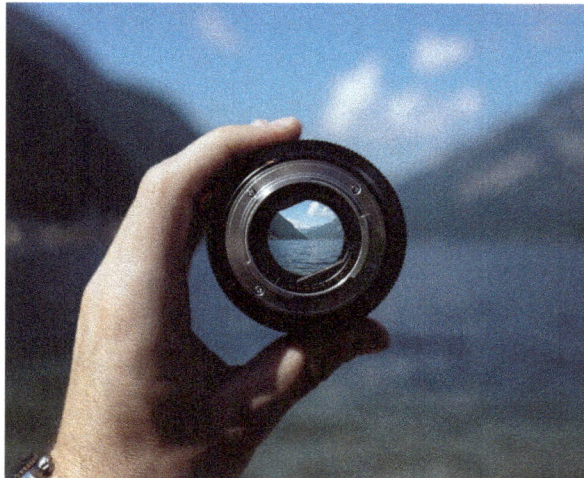

INTRODUCTION

Whole Food Plant Based eating is an evidence-based approach to creating health. It has been shown to:

Reduce Cholesterol

Reverse Type 2 Diabetes in many instances

Reduces Hypertension— normalize blood pressure

Ultimately reduce weight

As you will learn, the Standard American Diet (SAD) with its high content of fat, sugar, and salt is harmful to our health. A substantial amount of the health problems facing this nation can be traced to the detrimental effects of the Standard American Diet. Fast food has become so common that some busy individuals and families may consume fast food two or more times per day. Fast foods typically have higher proportions of fats, refined sugars, and salt than foods prepared thoughtfully with healthy nourishment in mind.

Many people have not grown up in households where cooking and meal preparation was a centerpiece of home life. Countless times I have heard comments like, "I don't cook!" or "By the time I get home, I am too tired to spend time in the kitchen cooking." For tens of thousands of years meal preparation and the sharing of a meal have been a primary activity that brought people together. We use phrases like hearth & home in recognition of the intimate connection between the two. However, we have lost our connection to where our food comes from and the joy it brings when we share a meal with others.

The staff of Wellness Weigh™ are here to support you through your journey and to empower you through education, reflection, breathing practice, and exercise. We will be helping you monitor your progress. At the end of the twelve weeks we hope you will have the tools you need to continue making healthful choices for the rest of your life.

Embrace the next twelve weeks knowing that everything you need to make changes is already within you. Trust that your body and the foods that you eat will make change possible.

Embrace the change coming your way.
Grow in new directions.
Explore, discover, reach and risk.
Change creates an energy inside of you
that you didn't realize you had.

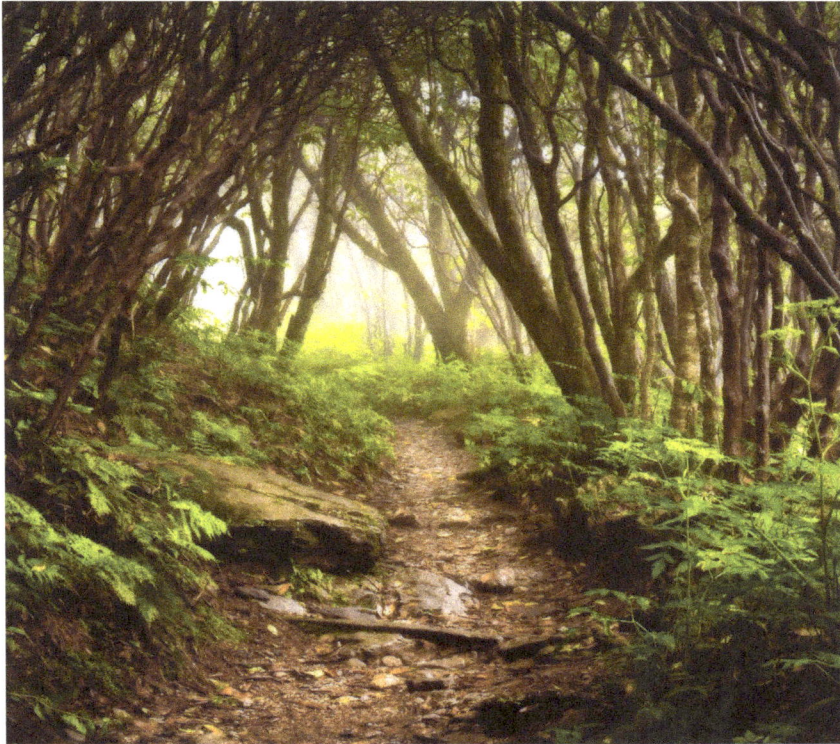

Week

1

Vital signs will be done weekly and will include:
blood pressure, pulse, weight, and abdominal circumference

Review the questionnaire and the consent form

Introduction to the Wellness Weigh™ program; a Wellness Weigh™ booklet
and 21-day Kickstart book will be distributed

Introduction to the Power Plate concept

Watch the first DVD from Food For Life, "Power of Your Plate"

Fasting lab work performed

Begin using the section for journaling (weekly)

Make a list of your current favorite foods and why they are your favorites

Set short-term and long-term goals

List support system at home and work

Food journal in the back of the booklet

Challenges/Solutions

_____

_____

_____

Make a list of your favorite foods and why they are your favorites

_____

_____

_____

Set short-term and long-term goals

_____

_____

_____

Make a list of the people who are part of your support system (at home & work)

_____

_____

_____

Reflections

_____

_____

_____

"Water is the Driving Force of all of Nature."

~ Leonardo da Vinci

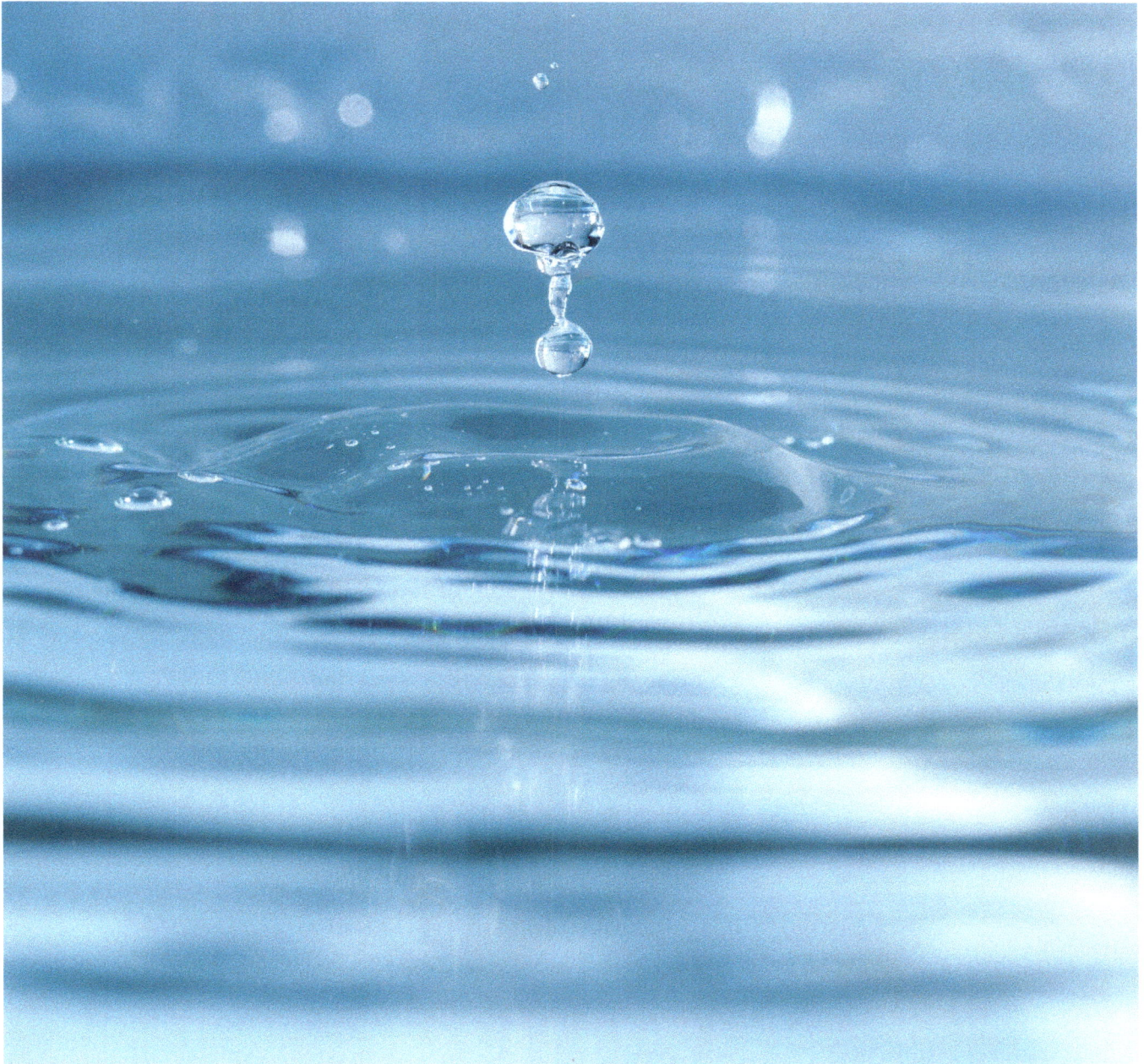

Vital signs will be done weekly and will include:
blood pressure, pulse, weight, and abdominal circumference

Review labs and goals

Develop a plan on how to institute the changes you intend to make

Start making changes
(think about small changes you can leverage for bigger changes)

Watch the second DVD from Food for Life, "Let's Go!"
(Questions & Answers)

Focus on drinking 32 ounces of water a day

Challenges/Solutions

Impressions from viewing the DVD

Make a plan about the changes you intend to make

What small changes can you leverage to achieve bigger changes?

What's it been like to remember to drink water? (32 ounces/day)

More Reflections

Your speed doesn't matter, forward is forward.

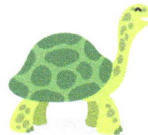

Eat Less From A Box
and More From the Earth.

"There are far better things ahead than any we leave behind."

~ C.S. Lewis

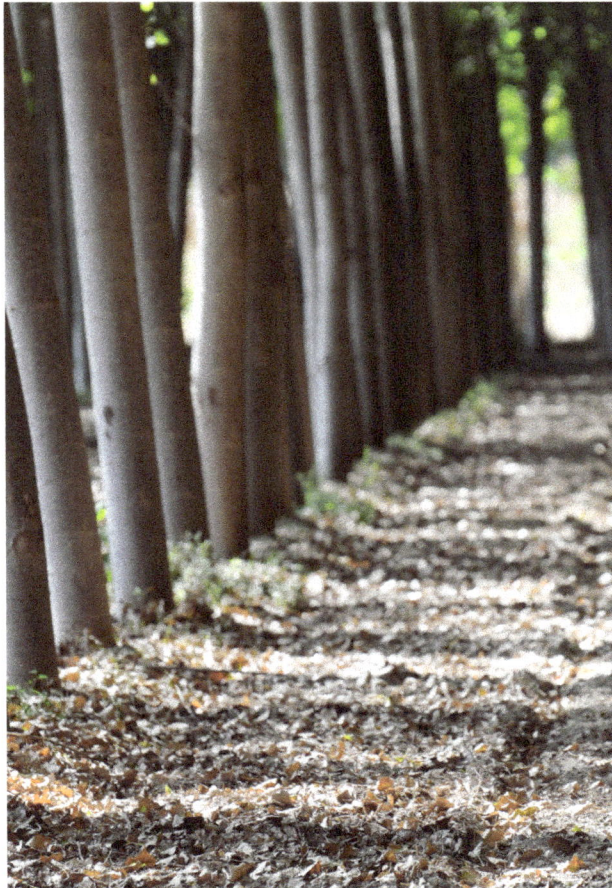

Vital signs will be done weekly and will include:
blood pressure, pulse, weight, and abdominal circumference

Meet with staff and begin menu planning

Art of reading labels. You will pay attention to ingredients and Nutritional Facts

---

The keys to menu planning

Eliminate sugar and refined carbohydrates

Clean out your cupboards and pantry

Challenges/Solutions

_____

_____

_____

Record the Carbohydrate, Fat, Sodium content of your favorite salsa or condiment (Ketchup, Mayonnaise, Mustard)

_____

_____

How did you feel as you discarded items from your cupboard?

_____

_____

More Reflections

_____

_____

_____

_____

Physical Hunger	vs	Emotional Hunger
Comes on gradual and can be postponed		Comes on suddenly and feels urgent
Can be satisfied with any type of food		Causes specific cravings like pizza, chocolate, & ice-cream
Once you are full you can stop eating		Tend to eat more than you normally would; eat until you feel uncomfortable
Causes satisfaction & does not cause guilt		Leaves you feeling guilty and cross with yourself

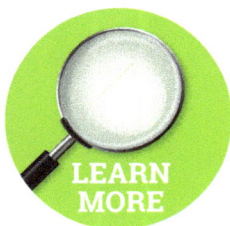

LEARN MORE

Here is an article on the seven types of hunger from The Mindfulness Project website.

londonmindful.com/blog/understanding-the-seven-types-of-hunger/

Dear Stress,
Let's break up.

Vital signs will be done weekly and will include:
blood pressure, pulse, weight, and abdominal circumference

Check in about how you are doing

Address some challenges that you need to troubleshoot

Review the types of hunger

Journal on the types of hunger that you experience during the week

Try a new veggie or fruit you have never eaten
(or decided you never liked) in a new recipe

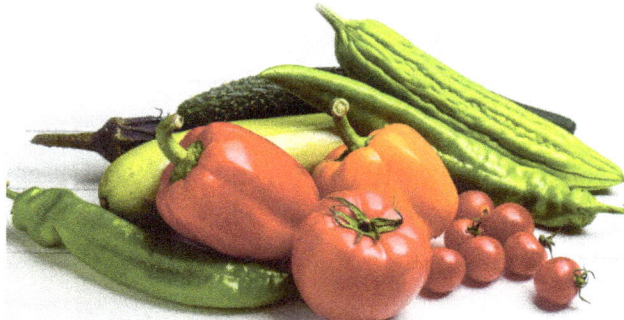

Challenges/Solutions

_____

_____

_____

What types of hunger did you experience during the week?

_____

_____

_____

What new fruit or vegetable did you try? What did you think of it?

_____

_____

_____

More Reflections

_____

_____

_____

"Movement is the song
of the body."

~ Vanda Scaravelli

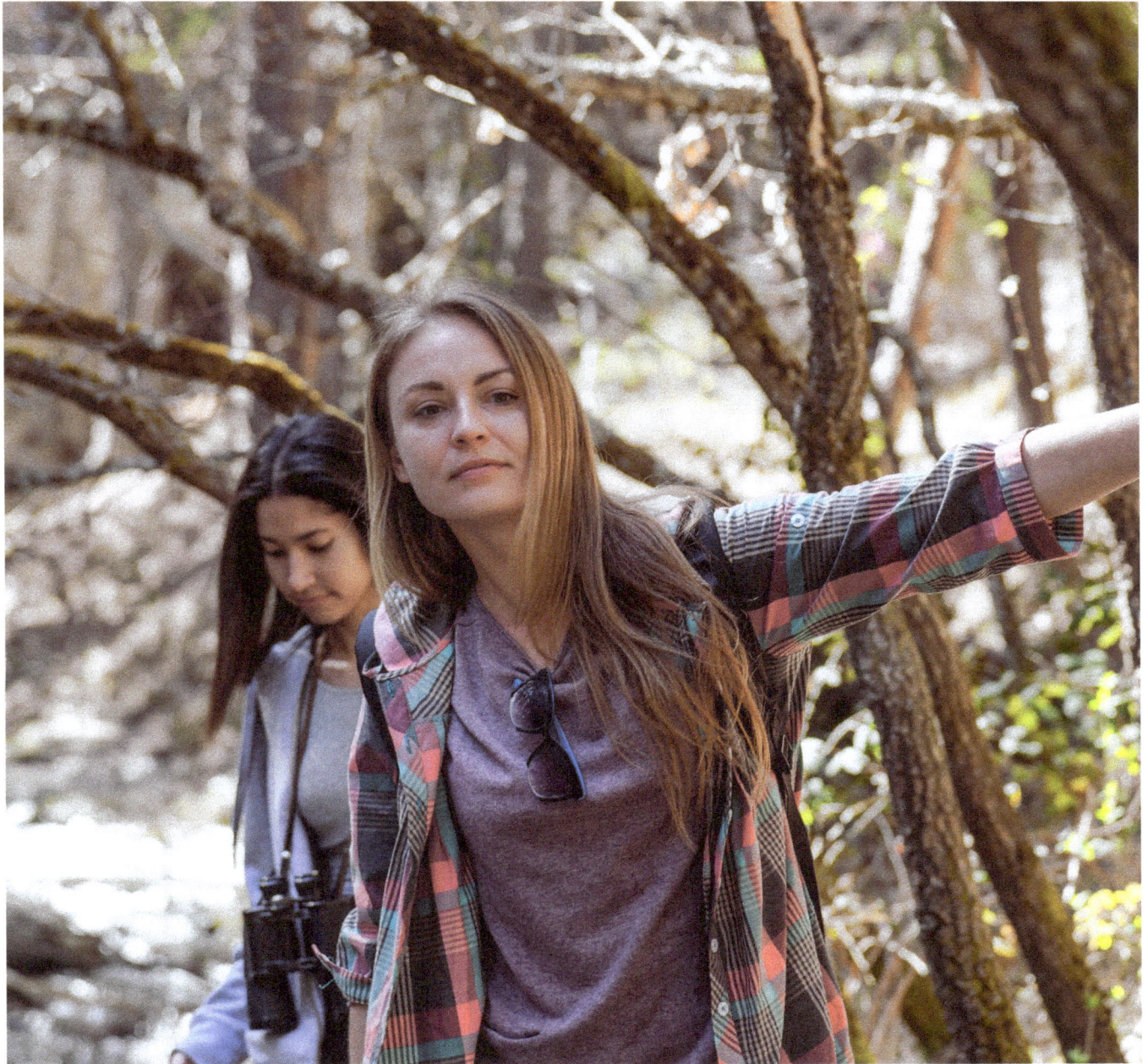

**Vital signs will be done weekly and will include:
blood pressure, pulse, weight, and abdominal circumference**

Watch the third DVD from Food for Life, "Getting in Gear"

Review goals

**Review the information about the importance of movement
for maintaining good health**

**Troubleshoot any physical limitations and time constraints
you are facing regarding movement and activity**

**Record your movement during the week and the feelings
you experience about movement**

**The Centers for Disease Control established that 10 min intervals of exercise three times
per day provides the same life extension benefits as 30 min of continuous exercise**

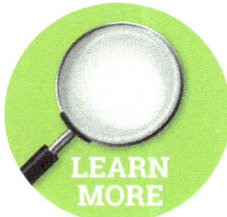

**LEARN
MORE**

Resources:

"Yoga for Weight Loss?" from WebMD
webmd.com/fitness-exercise/features/yoga-for-weight-loss#1

"How Exercise Helps You Lose Weight" from Healthline
healthline.com/health/diet-and-weight-loss-fitness-exercise

Challenges/Solutions

_____

_____

_____

What sort of movement/activity did you engage in & how did you feel about this?

_____

_____

_____

Write about your feelings regarding the movement/activities for the week

_____

_____

_____

More Reflections

_____

_____

_____

_____

Breathe in inspiration
and trust yourself;
the answer is YES
you can!

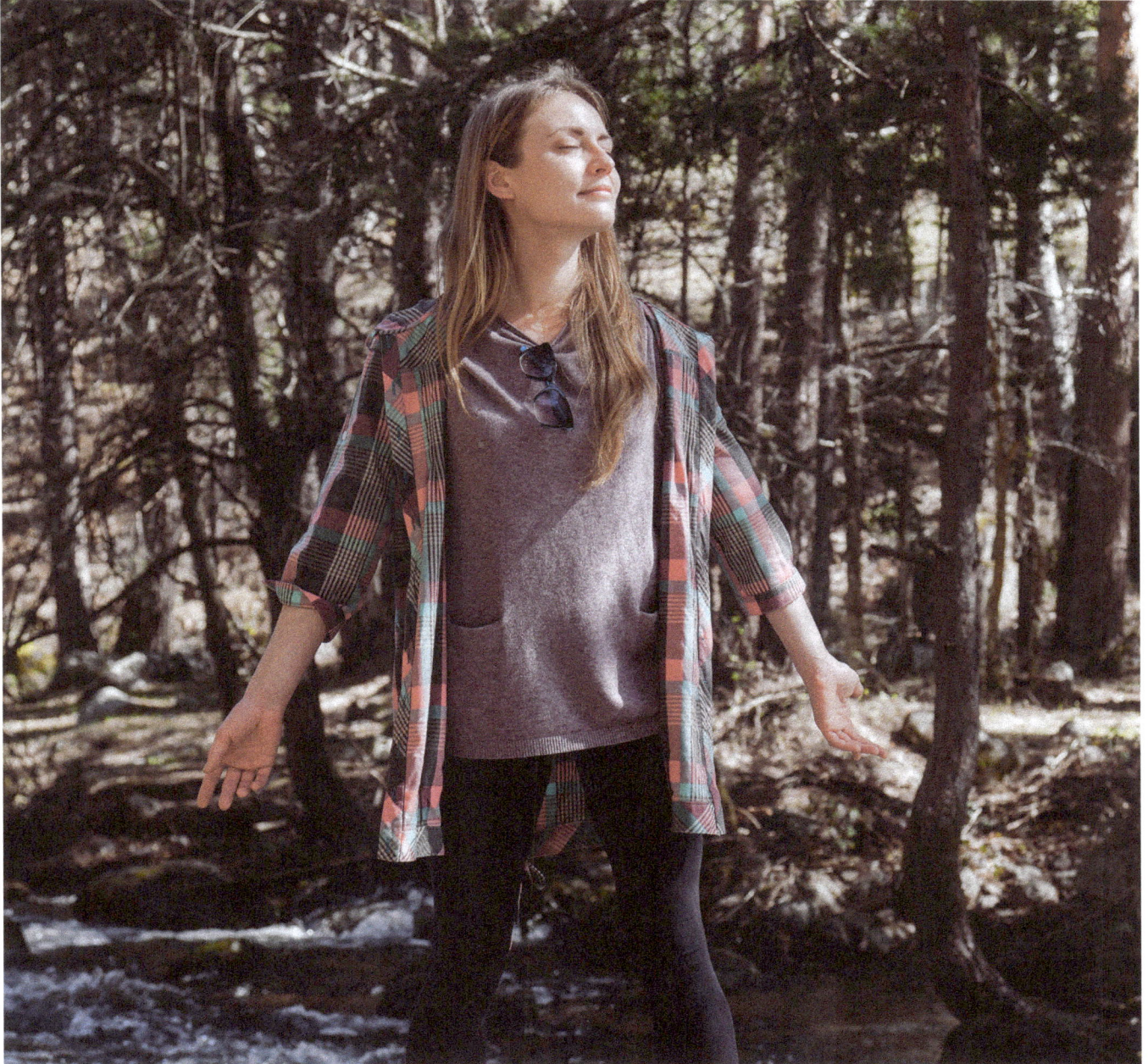

**Vital signs will be done weekly and will include:
blood pressure, pulse, weight, and abdominal circumference**

Resources for the home will be reviewed

Meet with staff to introduce breathing and breathing practices

---

Practice breathing and record your thoughts, feelings, and subtle impressions arising as you practiced breathing exercises in your journal

---

See if you can pay attention to your breathing at various times during the week

Watch a baby at rest; their belly gently rises and falls as they perform diaphragmatic breathing. Notice how most adults breath in more shallow, rapid fashion in which the chest rises and falls. With practice, we can learn to regulate our breath in order to harness profound health benefits.

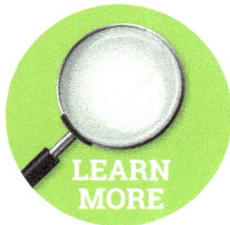

LEARN MORE

Guided Introduction to Abdominal Breathing

Here is a beautiful YouTube video offered by the City of Hope Cancer Treatment Centers. It is a gentle, guided five-minute introduction to abdominal breathing with beautiful images. **youtube.com/watch?v=bvdzTs0m510**

Relaxation Techniques

This is an article from Harvard Health Publications "Relaxation techniques: Breath control helps quell errant stress response"

health.harvard.edu/mind-and-mood/relaxation-techniques-breath-control-helps-quell-errant-stress-response

Challenges/Solutions

What changes or subtleties did you notice during your breathing practice?

Physical

Emotional

Spiritual

When did you find it helpful or challenging?

More Reflections

Let yourself rest.

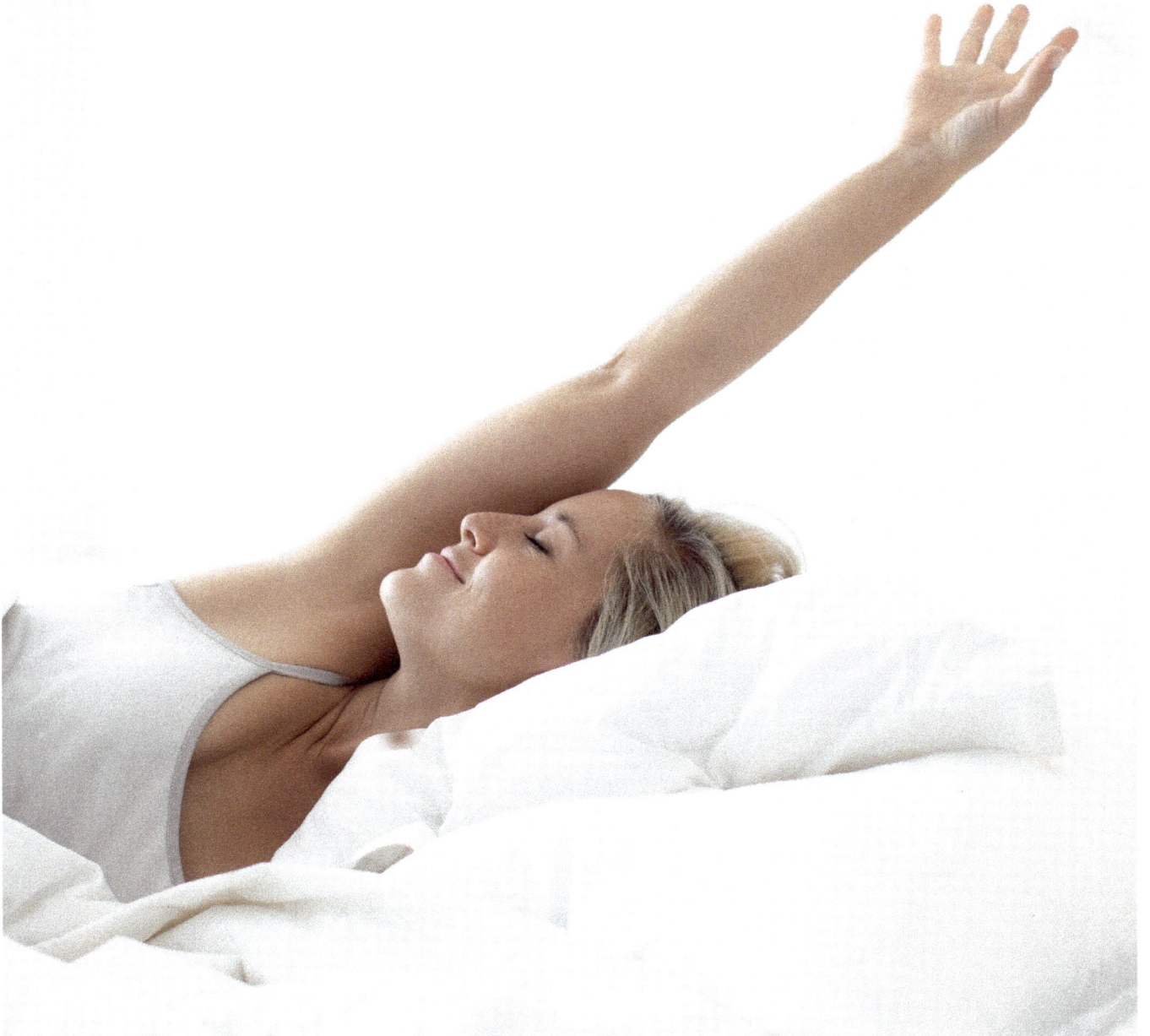

Vital signs will be done weekly and will include:
blood pressure, pulse, weight, and abdominal circumference

Watch the fourth DVD from Food for Life, "Breaking the Food Seduction"

Review handout(s) on the importance of rest and sleep and supplements

---

Record your sleep and periods of rest throughout the week

Insufficient sleep is linked to several diseases including heart disease and heart attacks, diabetes, obesity, and increases the likelihood of accidents and mood complaints. Among other things, sleep is a time when our bodies undergo repair and restoration of tissues that suffer wear and tear during the day.

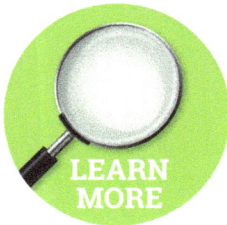

LEARN MORE

Resources:

"Why is Sleep Important?" from the National Institute of Health
nhlbi.nih.gov/health/health-topics/topics/sdd/why#

"Sleep More, Weigh Less" from WebMD
webmd.com/diet/sleep-and-weight-loss#1

Challenges/Solutions

_____
_____
_____

Record your impressions about the DVD

_____
_____
_____

Record your sleep for each night of the week. How did the amount of sleep affect you?

_____
_____
_____

More Reflections

_____
_____
_____

"Acupuncture works by restoring balance and triggering the body's natural response."

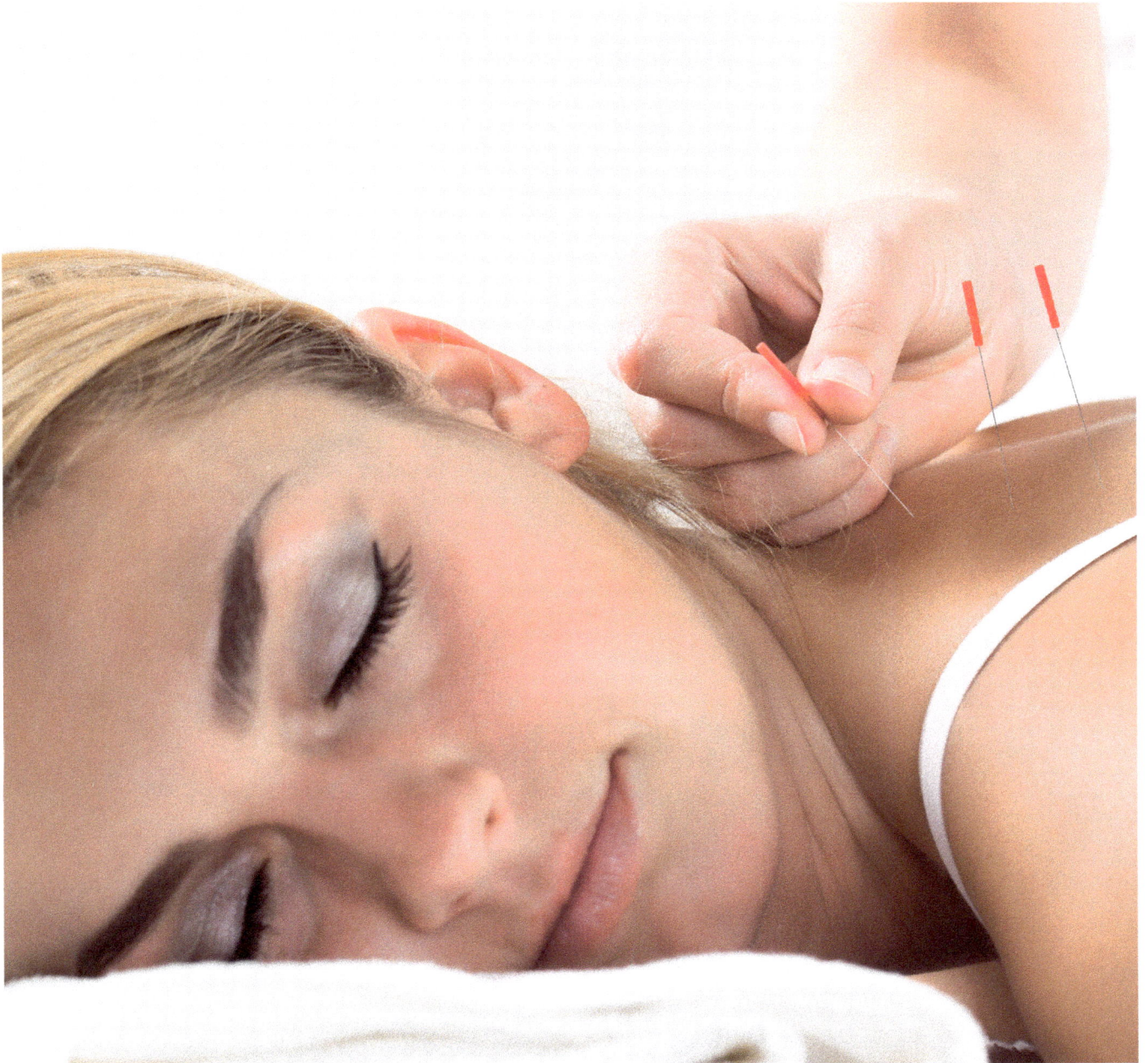

Vital signs will be done weekly and will include:
blood pressure, pulse, weight, and abdominal circumference

Meet with acupuncturist

Explore the Relaxation Response;
receive instruction on how to relax

Listen to your body

Help your body adjust to the changes in your routine and changes
in your nutrition that you've introduced

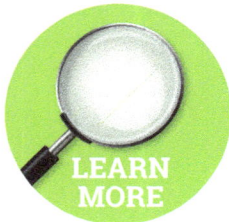

LEARN MORE

Acupuncture

"How Acupuncture Can relieve Pain and Improve Sleep, Digestion and Emotional Well Being" from University of California San Diego
cim.ucsd.edu/clinical-care/acupuncture.shtml

Gratitude

"Boost Your Health With a Dose of Gratitude" from WebMD
webmd.com/women/features/gratitute-health-boost#1

Challenges/Solutions

How were you able to implement relaxation during the week?

What brings you relaxation? How will you incorporate (or have you incorporated) some form of relaxation into your daily routines?

More Reflections

"I took a walk in the woods and came out taller than the trees"
~ Henry David Thoreau

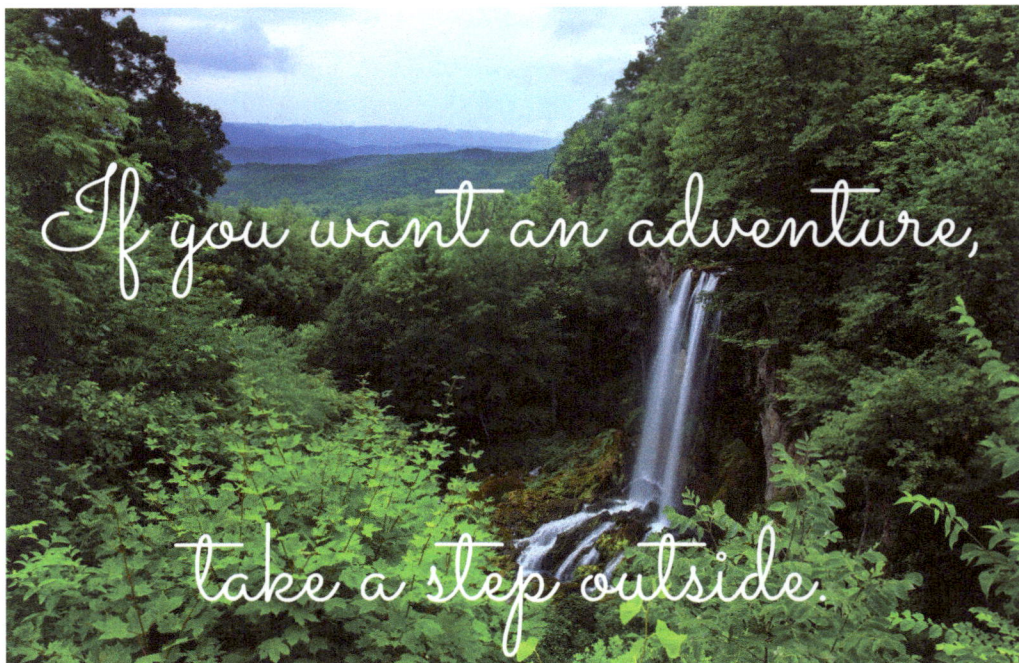

Photo by ForestWander.com

If you want an adventure, take a step outside.

"Of all the paths you take in life, make sure a few of them are in the dirt"
~ John Muir

Go play outside!

Start each day
with a grateful heart.

"Gratitude:
It's not happiness that brings us gratitude
it's gratitude that brings us happiness"

Vital signs will be done weekly and will include:
blood pressure, pulse, weight, and abdominal circumference

Watch the fifth DVD from Food for Life, "Keys for Natural Appetite Control"

The importance of cultivating positive emotions

Discussion on the importance of gratitude

Write down in your journal things for which you are grateful

Go outdoors and write your thoughts, reflections,
and impressions in your journal

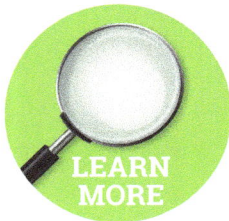

Resources:

"In Praise of Gratitude" from Harvard Newsletter
health.harvard.edu/newsletter_article/in-praise-of-gratitude

Here's Proof That Going Outside Makes You Healthier"
From Huffington Post
huffingtonpost.com/2014/06/22/how-the-outdoors-make-you_n_5508964.html

Challenges/Solutions

Record in your journal things for which you are grateful

Go outdoors and write your thoughts, reflections, and impressions in your journal

More Reflections

Nothing
Brings People together
like Good Food.

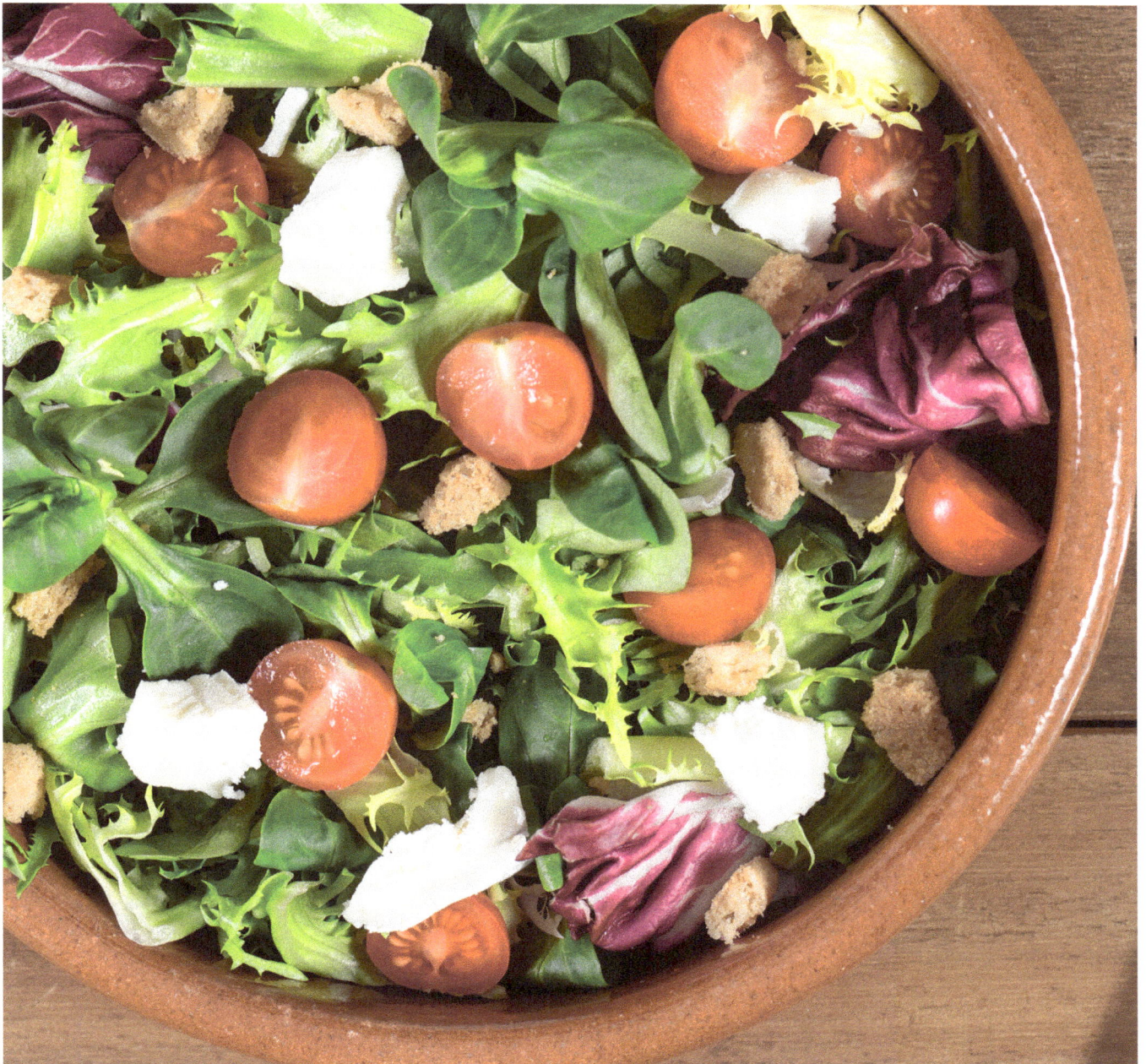

Vital signs will be done weekly and will include:
blood pressure, pulse, weight, and abdominal circumference.

Explore the concept of nourishing others

Prepare a recipe or some food you like and share it
with a co-worker, family member, or friend

Write down in your journal what it was like
to share food with someone else

Challenges/Solutions

_____

_____

_____

Record in your journal what it was like to feed and nourish another person

_____

_____

_____

How does eating alone differ for you from eating with someone else?

_____

_____

_____

More Reflections

_____

_____

_____

"Plan ahead and follow through"

"Planning is bringing the future into the present so that you can do something about it now."

– Alan Lakein

More **water**.

More **veggies**.

More **protein**.

More **cardio**.

More **strength**.

More **rest**.

More **sun**.

More happy and **fit**.

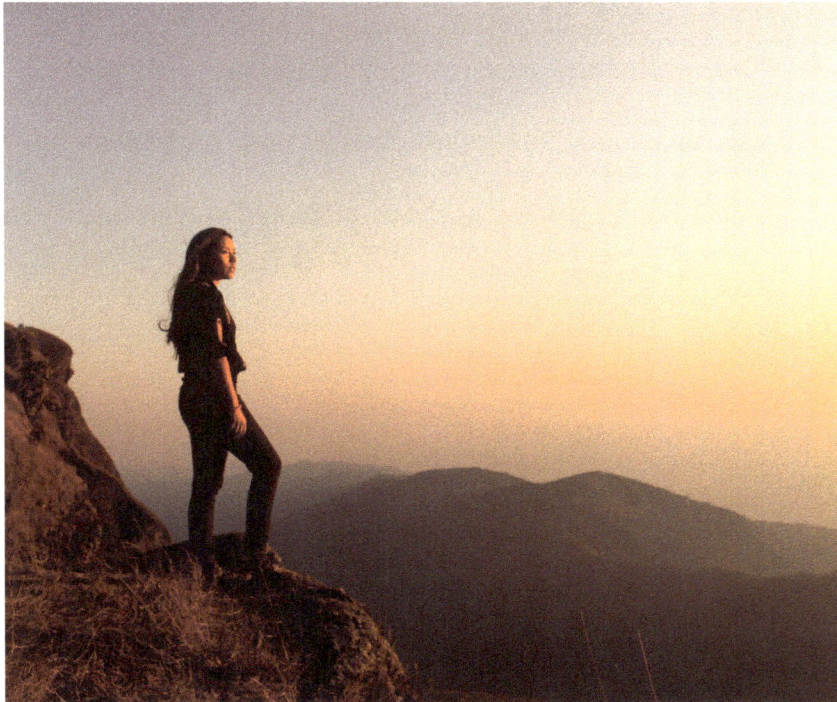

Week

11

Vital signs will be done weekly and will include:
blood pressure, pulse, weight, and abdominal circumference

Record your reflections on the goals you've attained
and those you intend to attain in the future

Fasting lab work will be obtained

Formulate a plan for the next steps you will take

Learn about monthly follow-up meetings and follow up

Join the Food for Life Facebook page and stay connected

facebook.com/Food-For-Life-369498683469323/

Challenges/Solutions

_____

_____

_____

Record in your journal your impressions concerning goals.

_____

_____

Imagine looking back to the past few months in one year, in five years, and in twenty years of having made significant changes in your lifestyle.

_____

_____

_____

More Reflections

_____

_____

_____

"You are braver than you believe,
stronger than you seem,
and smarter than you think."

~ Winnie the Pooh

"Make time to celebrate your accomplishments,
no matter how big or small"

Vital signs will be done weekly
and will include: blood pressure, pulse,
weight, and abdominal circumference

Review lab work obtained in week eleven

Final check out conducted

Complete and return the survey

More Reflections

	Portion Sizes		
HAND SYMBOL	**EQUIVALENT**	**FOODS**	**CALORIES**
	Fist 1 cup	Rice, pasta Fruit Veggies	200 75 40
	Palm 3 ounces	Meat Fish Poultry	160 160 160
	Handful 1 ounce	Nuts Raisins	170 85
	2 Handfuls 1 ounce	Chips Popcorn Pretzels	150 120 100
	Thumb 1 ounce	Peanut butter Hard cheese	170 100
	Thumb Tip 1 teaspoon	Cooking oil Mayonnaise, butter Sugar	40 35 15

Volume Conversions

60 drops = 1 teaspoon (5 ml)		4 tablespoons = 1/4 cup (60 ml)
16 dashes = 1 teaspoon (5 ml)		2 2/3 fluid ounces = 1/3 cup (80 ml)
8 pinches = 1 teaspoon (5 ml)		4 fluid ounces = 1/2 cup (120 ml)
1 1/2 teaspoons = 1/2 tablespoon (7.5 ml)		8 fluid ounces = 1 cup (240 ml)
3 teaspoons = 1 tablespoon (15 ml)		2 cups = 1 pint (475 ml)
2 tablespoons = 1 fluid ounce (30 ml)		4 cups = 1 quart (950 ml)

	Week 1	Week 2	Week 3	Week 4	Week 5	Week 6
BP						
Pulse						
Weight						
Abd. Circle						
Body Comp						
Body Fat %						
Bone Mass						
Body Water						
Visceral Fat						
Triglycerides						
Total Chol						
HDL						
LDL						
Glucose						

WELLNESS WEIGH™ Vital Signs Chart

	Week 7	Week 8	Week 9	Week 10	Week 11	Week 12
BP						
Pulse						
Weight						
Abd. Circle						
Body Comp						
Body Fat %						
Bone Mass						
Body Water						
Visceral Fat						
Triglycerides						
Total Chol						
HDL						
LDL						
Glucose						

WELLNESS WEIGH™ Vital Signs Chart

Food & Exercise Log

MEAL	MONDAY	TUESDAY	WEDNESDAY	THURSDAY	FRIDAY	SATURDAY	SUNDAY
Breakfast							
Lunch							
Dinner							
Snacks							
Water							

EXERCISE	MONDAY	TUESDAY	WEDNESDAY	THURSDAY	FRIDAY	SATURDAY	SUNDAY
Cardio							
Strength							
Min/Day							

Food & Exercise Log

MEAL	MONDAY	TUESDAY	WEDNESDAY	THURSDAY	FRIDAY	SATURDAY	SUNDAY
Breakfast							
Lunch							
Dinner							
Snacks							
Water							

EXERCISE	MONDAY	TUESDAY	WEDNESDAY	THURSDAY	FRIDAY	SATURDAY	SUNDAY
Cardio							
Strength							
Min/Day							

Food & Exercise Log							
MEAL	**MONDAY**	**TUESDAY**	**WEDNESDAY**	**THURSDAY**	**FRIDAY**	**SATURDAY**	**SUNDAY**
Breakfast							
Lunch							
Dinner							
Snacks							
Water							

EXERCISE	**MONDAY**	**TUESDAY**	**WEDNESDAY**	**THURSDAY**	**FRIDAY**	**SATURDAY**	**SUNDAY**
Cardio							
Strength							
Min/Day							

Food & Exercise Log

MEAL	MONDAY	TUESDAY	WEDNESDAY	THURSDAY	FRIDAY	SATURDAY	SUNDAY
Breakfast							
Lunch							
Dinner							
Snacks							
Water							

EXERCISE	MONDAY	TUESDAY	WEDNESDAY	THURSDAY	FRIDAY	SATURDAY	SUNDAY
Cardio							
Strength							
Min/Day							

Food & Exercise Log

MEAL	MONDAY	TUESDAY	WEDNESDAY	THURSDAY	FRIDAY	SATURDAY	SUNDAY
Breakfast							
Lunch							
Dinner							
Snacks							
Water							

EXERCISE	MONDAY	TUESDAY	WEDNESDAY	THURSDAY	FRIDAY	SATURDAY	SUNDAY
Cardio							
Strength							
Min/Day							

Food & Exercise Log

MEAL	MONDAY	TUESDAY	WEDNESDAY	THURSDAY	FRIDAY	SATURDAY	SUNDAY
Breakfast							
Lunch							
Dinner							
Snacks							
Water							

EXERCISE	MONDAY	TUESDAY	WEDNESDAY	THURSDAY	FRIDAY	SATURDAY	SUNDAY
Cardio							
Strength							
Min/Day							

Food & Exercise Log

MEAL	MONDAY	TUESDAY	WEDNESDAY	THURSDAY	FRIDAY	SATURDAY	SUNDAY
Breakfast							
Lunch							
Dinner							
Snacks							
Water							

EXERCISE	MONDAY	TUESDAY	WEDNESDAY	THURSDAY	FRIDAY	SATURDAY	SUNDAY
Cardio							
Strength							
Min/Day							

Food & Exercise Log

MEAL	MONDAY	TUESDAY	WEDNESDAY	THURSDAY	FRIDAY	SATURDAY	SUNDAY
Breakfast							
Lunch							
Dinner							
Snacks							
Water							

EXERCISE	MONDAY	TUESDAY	WEDNESDAY	THURSDAY	FRIDAY	SATURDAY	SUNDAY
Cardio							
Strength							
Min/Day							

Food & Exercise Log

MEAL	MONDAY	TUESDAY	WEDNESDAY	THURSDAY	FRIDAY	SATURDAY	SUNDAY
Breakfast							
Lunch							
Dinner							
Snacks							
Water							

EXERCISE	MONDAY	TUESDAY	WEDNESDAY	THURSDAY	FRIDAY	SATURDAY	SUNDAY
Cardio							
Strength							
Min/Day							

Food & Exercise Log

MEAL	MONDAY	TUESDAY	WEDNESDAY	THURSDAY	FRIDAY	SATURDAY	SUNDAY
Breakfast							
Lunch							
Dinner							
Snacks							
Water							

EXERCISE	MONDAY	TUESDAY	WEDNESDAY	THURSDAY	FRIDAY	SATURDAY	SUNDAY
Cardio							
Strength							
Min/Day							

Food & Exercise Log

MEAL	MONDAY	TUESDAY	WEDNESDAY	THURSDAY	FRIDAY	SATURDAY	SUNDAY
Breakfast							
Lunch							
Dinner							
Snacks							
Water							

EXERCISE	MONDAY	TUESDAY	WEDNESDAY	THURSDAY	FRIDAY	SATURDAY	SUNDAY
Cardio							
Strength							
Min/Day							

Food & Exercise Log

MEAL	MONDAY	TUESDAY	WEDNESDAY	THURSDAY	FRIDAY	SATURDAY	SUNDAY
Breakfast							
Lunch							
Dinner							
Snacks							
Water							

EXERCISE	MONDAY	TUESDAY	WEDNESDAY	THURSDAY	FRIDAY	SATURDAY	SUNDAY
Cardio							
Strength							
Min/Day							

www.ingramcontent.com/pod-product-compliance
Lightning Source LLC
Chambersburg PA
CBHW041430270326
41934CB00020B/3489